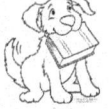

Undetected - Unchecked Health Issued
A Guide To Better Health

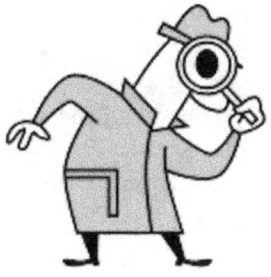

K. B. LeMere, ND
Author

Health by Design Publishing
Dallas, Texas

I am blessed to have three loving men in my life:

My husband for the countless hours of time together he has given up,

My son for his encouragement to press on,

My father who taught me I can do anything through Christ that strengths me.

This book is dedicated to them.

Undetected Unchecked Health Issues
A Guide To Better Health

Copyright © 2016

K. B. LeMere ND

E-book

Health by Design Publishing

Author Information

Email: drklemere@gmail.com

Web: www.author-kblemere.com

Book in Print

ISBN 9781543285017

9 781543 285017

Printed in the United States of America

Contents

UNDETECTED HEALTH ISSUES

Candida, Thrush, Candidiasis, Fungus

This little book is intended to give you knowledge and help you understand about the hidden health issues that could be the undetected health issue that most medical doctors do not check. Candida is a fungus that normally lives in a healthy balance with other bacteria and yeast in the body.

- ***Candida*** *is defined as a yeastlike parasitic fungus that can sometimes cause thrush.*

- ***Thrush*** *is defined as an infection of the mouth and throat by a yeastlike fungus, causing whitish patches.*

- ***Candidiasis*** *is defined as an infection with candida, especially as causing oral or vaginal thrush.*

- ***Fungus*** *is defined as any group of unicellular, multicellular, or syncytial spore-producing organisms that feeds on yeastlike parasitic fungus.*

Certain conditions can cause any one of these to multiply, weakening the immune system and causing one of the infections. Symptoms often worsen in damp and/or moldy places, and/or after consumption of foods containing sugar, vinegar, and/or yeast. Systemic candidiasis is an overgrowth of Candida throughout the body. In the most severe cases, Candida can travel through the bloodstream to invade every system in the body, causing a type of blood poisoning called Candida septicemia. These conditions usually occur in persons with serious underlying illnesses.

Case studies done at Harvard Medical School, the natural remedies division, reported the following symptoms have improved, or been eliminated, by killing the overgrowth of the fungus in a person.

Example of Symptoms

Fatigue, unexplained tiredness
Chronic Fatigue (CFS)
Fibromyalgia (FMS)
Headaches
Depression and Manic Depression
Multiple Chemical Sensitivities, (Environmental Illness)
Asthma
Psoriasis
Cystitis
Sexual dysfunction (ED)
Infertility
Vaginal yeast Infections
Vulvar Burning
Endometriosis
Some Autoimmune Diseases
Children:
Ear disorders
ADHD
Improvements in Autism

Anyone, who has been on long-term antibiotic therapy or has taken antibiotics more than once a year, probably has an overgrowth of Candida in their body. Antibiotics weaken the immune system and destroy the "friendly" bacteria that normally keeps Candida under control. As Candida proliferates, it releases toxins that weaken the immune system further. By the time I see a client, they are so tired and fatigued he or she does not know what to do. Most medical doctors do not routinely check for a Candida imbalance. A simple blood test can determine if you have an overgrowth. If your blood test results come back with high amounts of Candida they usually fail to mention it. Alway ask for a copy of your blood test results. What can you do, start immediately taking probiotic to rebuild your intestinal balance.

The other two main factors that increase the chances of contracting the infection, Candidiasis, are pregnancy or the use of corticosteroid drugs. If you must take antibiotics or corticosteroid drugs, avoid getting Candida by taking "Healthy Trinity" by Natrin or any combination of probiotics which produce good bacteria back into the body. Only take the freeze-dried version of a probiotic if you can't find anything else.

Couples may have a challenge. If one partner has candida concealed in their blood stream, it can be passed sexually through intercourse or by saliva. Some of my female clients worked hard to get healthy, but could never get 100% because their partners would not follow the treatment plan. I had one client who had a really bad case; she had a skin rash and chronic fatigue so bad she could not do anything but lie on the couch all day. She followed my instructions to the letter and had an 85% recovery in three months, but she could not get to 100%. Her husband thought all this stuff was bunk. Once she abstained from physical contact, he agreed to follow the diet and take the pills. Her husband no longer thinks this is bunk: he enjoys the sexual relationship they now have and how great he feels.

In our country today, we have a serious candida problem that began years ago from taking extensive antibiotics, birth control pills, and steroids for infections. Also, in my practice, I have found people with mercury toxicity having high amounts of Candida. Mercury toxicity can come from old amalgam (silver) fillings in your teeth by leaking mercury into your body. Mercury salts inhibit the growth of the necessary "friendly" bacteria in the intestines. This allows the candida to colonize in the digestive tract causing problems in the entire body. The colonies produce toxins that are absorbed into the bloodstream which can affect the immune system, hormonal balances, and thought processes.

I have seen a pattern indicating that yeast related illnesses are a hidden cause for most autoimmune diseases. Ninety-five percent of clients with Hypothyroidism have Candida. The prescription drugs changes the balance in the intestinal tract, by killing the bacterium that keeps Candida in check. Now the fungus takes over.

The bully, a concealed fungus pushes its way into the intestinal lining destroying cells and brush borders. When I was diagnosed with Connective Tissue Disease my blood test showed high levels of Candida. My doctor ordered the blood test as part of my work up, but when she received the results, she did not even mention it to me. That is why it is important to always get a copy of your test results and learn to read them.

Medical Treatment vs Herbal

Medical treatment for Candidiasis involves the use of anti-fungal medications such as Nystatin, or Amphotericin B, which are anti-fungal medication used for serious fungal infections. Some of the fungal infections they are used to treat are aspergillosis, blastomycosis, candida, coccidioidomycosis, and cryptococcosis. For certain infections it is given with flucytosine. It is typically given by injection into a vein Common side effects include a reaction with fever, chills, and headaches soon after the medication is given, as well as kidney problems. Other serious side effects include low blood potassium and inflammation of the heart. Amphotericin B was originally made from *Streptomyces nodosus* in 1955. It is on the World Health Organization's List of Essential Medicines, the most effective and safe medicines needed in a health system.

Nystatin was discovered in 1950 by Rachel Fuller Brown and Elizabeth Lee Hazen. It is on the World Health Organization's List of Essential Medicines, the most effective and safe medicines needed in a health system. It is used to treat Candida infections of the skin including diaper rash, thrush, esophageal candidiasis, and vaginal yeast infections. It may also be used to prevent candidiasis in those who are at high risk. Nystatin may be used by mouth, in the vagina, or applied to the skin. Common side effects when applied to the skin include burning, itching, and a rash. Common side effects when taken by mouth include vomiting and diarrhea

It is prescribed as a standard drug for nail fungus. If you have nail fungus, then you already have fungus in your blood. To a naturopathic doctor, these drugs, especially if chronic or repeated, can lead to the development of stronger strains of yeast that are drug resistant. Higher dosages are then required which in turn further weaken the immune system. You can use a topical anti-fungal, such as oregano or tea tree oil on the nail surface to kill the fungus. It is best to work from the inside of the body to the outside. There are several natural remedies that work. They do require taking a product along with diet control and topical applications to eliminate the fungus. The product depends on the seriousness of your condition.

Herbal supplements will attack and kill it. The herb tea Pau d'Arco contains an antibacterial and anti-fungal agent, however, it does have an alkaloid base, so some people may not benefit from its use. This tea has a bitter taste, but you can alternate between Pau d'Arco tea and clover tea or mix them together. You can use Stevia to sweeten. You can buy these in the grocery or herb store. Tea is a good aid to assist herbal supplement, but will not kill the fungus by itself.

Many clients, especially those with thyroid disease, can be prone to persistent Candida or resistant strains that develop rapidly due to genetic mutation. Two herbal products are on the top of my list.

1.***Nature's Secret Candistroy Kit***. It is a 2 part program to support yeast balance, promote healthy intestinal flora and replenish good bacteria. Candistroy is a comprehensive, all-natural system that helps the body rid itself of fungus and replenishes good bacteria. It contains a unique proprietary blend of zinc tannates, berberine-containing herbs, digestive bitters and beneficial bacteria as well as F.O.S. and NAG that have been proven to help enhance the proliferation of your beneficial bacteria in both the small and large intestines. It can be purchased at Whole Foods market or ordered online for $15.00 a box on Amazon, 60 tablets. You should plan to take 3-4 boxes. This product is not a harsh product, but is a good place to start.

2.Raintree's A-F Anti-Fungal is a 650 mg formula from raintree.com online only. It is a synergistic blend of herbs from the rain forest of: jatoba, Brazilian Peppertree, Anamu, Bellaco Capsi, Matico, Piri-piri, Pau d'arco, Ubos, Fedegoso, Tamamuri, Guaco, and Graviola. $ 29.95 for 120 capsules. Recommended daily to start with 2 capsules 3 times a day for the first week, then 2 capsules twice a day for 90 days. Must be used in conjunction with a probiotic and special nutrition plan. This is the most expensive and require purchasing a probiotic separately, but it is the most powerful.

Many clients ask me if they can take Colloidal silver, it is a natural broad-spectrum antiseptic that fights infection, subdues inflammation, and promotes healing, but will not eliminate Candida by itself. Unfortunately, no matter what you take, it is a

90 day process with fatigue symptoms for the first three weeks. It only takes four easy steps.

Step One: Take supplements to kill candida and

Step Two: Eliminate the fungus from the inside out take care of your colon

Step Three: Flush it out with water

Step Four: A special nutrition plan

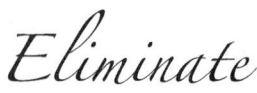 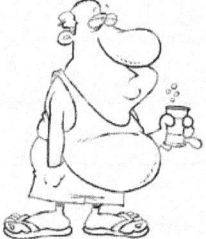

The intestinal system is comprised of the lower bowel, known as the colon or large intestine, and the rectum. The colon may be divided into three parts: ascending, transverse, and descending. It is only five feet long, but it has a 2 1/2 inch diameter, three times the diameter of the small intestine. The colon forms a frame for the convoluted shape of the small intestine.

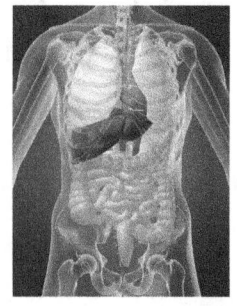 The function of the intestinal system is to absorb and remove waste products from the body so they will be excreted and not reabsorbed. The colon helps to eliminate food that cannot be digested, along with bacteria, parasites, and waste. Problems with the colon are frequently due to a poor diet. Two things can be done to strengthen the colon, (a) improve the diet and (b) periodically cleanse the colon. This program will cleanse the colon and remove the candida that has died off and not being eliminated.

When the colon is flooded with junk food, the body cannot properly handle the waste. This waste may lodge in colon pockets and if not removed, the waste may recycle into the bloodstream.

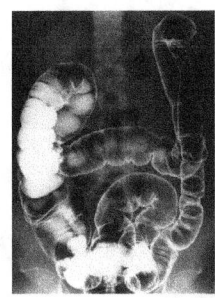 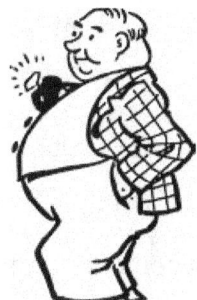

CONSTIPATION is a common problem characterized by sluggish colon action. It may be caused by eating highly refined foods, eating too quickly, having a stressful lifestyle, or failing to exercise adequately. Mucus-forming foods are especially prone to contribute to constipation. These foods may form a sticky matter that adheres to the colon wall. This attracts further buildup, that block absorption of minerals and traps toxins. A stagnant bowel may lead to constipation, allowing toxins to spread throughout the body.

Fiber

One way to alleviate constipation and other colon problems is to add fiber to the daily diet. Bowel activity is affected by the amount of fiber, as well as water, present in the colon. In general, fiber includes such foods as whole grains, fruits, vegetables, and beans. Fruits and vegetables are known as cleansing foods. Cultures who have a diet of vegetables and whole grains do not have problems with constipation, colon cancer, diverticulitis, or other associated problems. The high fiber content aids in the proper elimination of body waste.

There are two types of fiber, soluble and insoluble. Each type performs a different role. Soluble fiber forms a gel with water, creating a laxative effect. Soluble fiber traps sugar and cholesterol. Pectin, gum, and mucilage are examples of soluble fibers and can be found in wheat, corn bran, and cereal grains. Sponge-like insoluble fiber contributes to regular bowel function by adding bulk. Fruits, vegetables, beans, and oats contain insoluble fibers such as cellulose, hemicellulose, and lignin.

Fiber also helps to absorb and thus eliminate toxic substances. Of course, bran is an excellent source of dietary fiber. When adding bran to your diet, begin with a small amount, such as 1 tsp. per day. As the body becomes accustomed to bran, increase the amount of your daily intake.

Acidophilus bacteria also contribute to a healthy colon by supplying friendly bacteria that assist in colon function. Simply changing eating habits is not enough to achieve a healthy colon. First the colon must be fully cleansed.

Over the years of practice I saw many people that do not make elimination a priority daily. One man said he only eliminates once a month, another man said, Oh, I usually go about every three months! Really? The result can be spotted in their physical appearance.

The first comment I hear as we discuss the elimination process is - Laxatives are dangerous. My answer is always, not eliminating is far more dangerous. I suggest a herbal product called "Reneu" from an international company in Dallas called FirstFitness Nutrition.

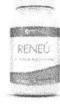 Reneu is described as a inner body and colon cleanse. It supports cleansing and detoxification of the inner body and colon to help enhance the

absorption of food, vitamins and minerals, promote good health, and optimize weight loss. It can be ordered online at firstfitness.com. It is not a laxative but a stool softener made from wild cherry bark. When taken every night before bed you will eliminate naturally in the morning without any trouble.

Flush it out!

Water is used in our bodily fluid components for blood, lymph, digestive juice, urine, tears, and sweat. In addition, water is used in bodily components for circulation, digestion, absorption, and elimination. Water carries the electrolytes and mineral salts that help convey electrical currents in the body. The mineral salts in most water are sodium, potassium, calcium, magnesium, and chloride.

Every day our bodies loses 8 lbs. of fluid

2 pounds - Skin - sweat
2 pounds. - Lungs - exhaling
2 pounds - Kidney - urine
2 pounds - Bowel - elimination

You must drink 64 ounces of water a day to replenished the two quarts of water our bodies use. Water is also used for our bodily functions: Circulation, digestion, absorption, and elimination. More importantly, water carries the electrolytes and mineral salts that help convey electrical currents in the body. The mineral salts are sodium, potassium, calcium, magnesium, and chloride.

Tap Water: There are 3 advantages of using tap water. 1) convenience 2)available 3)it costs only pennies, but; tap water has many health disadvantages. The water is process in a treatment plant in settling tanks, which filters through sand and gravel. This does not completely make the water pure for drinking. The chemicals used for purification may not clear all the environmental pollutants that contaminate our water. If you must drink tap water, use a filter. Most modern refrigerators have filtration systems.

Spring Water: Drink 64 ounces of spring water a day to replenished the two quarts of water our bodies use. Water is used to maintain our bodily fluids components made up of : blood, lymph, digestive juice, urine, tears and sweat. Water is used for our bodily functions: circulation, digestion, absorption, and elimination. It is very importantly to note that water carries the electrolytes and mineral salts conveying electrical currents in the body. The mineral salts are: sodium, potassium, calcium, magnesium, and chloride.

Distilled Water: There are two schools of though concerning drinking distilled water. Some natural health practitioners feel it is the best and the cleanest water to drink because the distillation process removes all the minerals, organisms, and chemicals from the water, making it pure H20. Other practitioners feel the human body does not use these inorganic minerals. The majority feel by drinking distilled water you can become deficient in minerals. Many minerals that can be used in the body are in the inorganic or salt state and are not part of the organic tissue.

The best drinking water, according to my research, is Reverse Osmosis or Ozonated, which has a high oxygen level. Ozone therapy is a form of alternative medicine treatment that purports to increase the amount of oxygen in the body through the introduction of ozone.

The best way to drink water is in intervals throughout the day. Do not drink a 16 ounce full glass of water before or just after meals. This will dilute digestive juices and reduce food nutrient assimilation.

Water intervals:

      10:00 A.M. -2 cups/16 ounces

      1:00 P.M. - 2 cups/16 ounces

      3:00 P.M. - 2 cups/16 ounces

      5:00 P.M. - 2 cups/16 ounces

Don't drink more than a gallon of water a day, because it becomes a negative and will wash all the minerals out of your system. But if you are dehydrated from lack of water or drinking caffeine, then you need to replace what you have lost. If you drink any alcohol for every 8 ounces, you need to replenish your water level with 16 ounces of water. Alcohol is dehydrating and acidic. Flying on an airplane is very dehydrating. Drink bottled water before, during, and after the flight. It is a plus and minus system. For any minus beverage you drink (acidic's like soda or caffeine) you must add back in 16 ounces of water to equalize the fluids. So for every one glass of wine, soda, coffee you drink you have to drink one 16 ounce glass of water to create a balance.

The way to replenish the body's engine with water is to drink four 16-ounce glasses in a day, one glass every two hours. Add lemon to aid the body in alkalinity. Most of my clients are overwhelmed with this idea until I demonstrate by lining up four 16 ounce bottles of water. Once they see it they usually say, *"Oh, I can do that."* Do not drink a full glass of water with meals or just after meals. Drinking water with meals dilutes digestive juices, preventing the meal from being properly digested and hinders the assimilation cycles. *Do not* drink over a gallon a day unless you are dehydrated. A gallon a day will wash all the minerals out of your system. If you drink an alcohol based drink, for every 8 oz. of alcohol you must replenish the dehydration it causes with 16 ounces of water. Alcohol and flying are very dehydrating. Regular use of alcohol causes acidosis, a highly acidic condition. Herbal Teas are soothing and acidic, so you drink them with meals. Teas act as a diuretic and can cause dehydration, again balance with water intake.

Nutrition Plans

Follow the nutritional plan on the following pages to **kill** off the food source that feeds the candida.

Follow these guidelines while elimination of yeast is in progress:

- ☑ Eat vegetables, fish, and gluten–free grains such as brown rice and millet (see food plan)

- ☑ For vaginal candidiasis, apply plain unflavored yogurt directly to the vagina. This helps to inhibit the growth of the fungus

- ☑ For skin, rash and candidiasis break out on the skin use a topical essential oils, such as tea tree or oregano. If your skin is sensitive mix with olive oil.

- ☑ Take supplemental as described above. Acidophilus or bifidus to help to restore the normal balance of flora in the bowel and vagina. The best one is "Healthy Trinity" by Natren which can be ordered on Amazon. You can buy it at Whole Foods Grocery Stores or an herb store also. Do not let them talk you into anything else.

- ☑ Take some type of fiber daily. The best is Flax powder by Omega Life or *"Barlenes"* You can put it on your salad, smoothie, and oatmeal or in any food or cereal.

☑ Drink water as discussed earlier, a minimum 64 oz. daily. Measure it.

☑ Eat a diet that is fruit-free, sugar-free, and yeast-free. Candida thrives in a sugary environment, so your diet should be low in carbohydrates and contain no yeast products or sugar in any form, or anything that can turn into sugar in the body. You can use "Stevia" for a sweetener.

☑ **No** aged cheeses, alcohol, baked goods, chocolate, dried fruits, fermented foods, grains containing gluten (wheat, oats, rye, and barley), ham, honey, nut butters, pickles, potatoes, raw mushrooms, soy sauce, sprouts, or vinegar. These foods contain yeast.

☑ Eliminate citrus and acidic fruits if your ph is .6 or lower, (such as oranges, grapefruit, lemons, tomatoes, pineapple, and limes) from your diet for six weeks. Then add back only a few twice weekly. Note: these can be eaten if picked fresh.

☑ For constipation, use L-bifidus, a retention enema, or *Reneu*, an all natural herbal product, by First Fitness. You should have a bowel movement 3-4 times a day.

☑ Take only hypoallergenic supplements

☑ Prevent re-infection by replacing your toothbrush every thirty days.

☑ Wear white cotton underwear. Synthetic fibers lead to increased perspiration, which creates a hospitable environment for Candida. It traps bacteria, which can cause a secondary infection.

☑ Avoid household chemical products and cleaners, chlorinated water, mothballs, synthetic textiles, damp and moldy places.

Chronic or persistent candida after taking supplement for 30 days, might be a sign of immune system dysfunction. You body is providing an environment more conducive to the growth of yeast. If this is the case, add the herb Cat's Claw if you are not feeling a difference after 30 days.

Organize: Begin with cleaning and reorganizing your kitchen. Start with the pantry and then the refrigerator. The reason that you are going to get rid of the following foods and drinks is that they contain nutritionally deficient simple carbohydrates that encourage yeast overgrowth and promote poor health. To overcome Candida-related health problems you will need to remove these from your diet.

Get Rid Of: Sugar, corn syrup, white bread and other white flour products, sodas, ready to eat cereals, and all the sweet, fat snack foods, processed and prepared junk foods which have hydrogenated or partially hydrogenated fats, with food coloring and additives.

On the following pages you will find lists of:
- Food you **cannot** eat
- Food you can eat
- Meal suggestions
- Lifestyle "Do Not's" at a glance
- Eating out choices
- Supplement shopping
- Shopping list

The No No List at a Glance

Foods You CANNOT Eat – Anything that contains Sugar, Yeast, Vinegar, or Mildews

* Sugars - sucrose, fructose, maltose, lactose, glucose, mannitol, sorbitol, galactose, maple sugar, maple syrup, brown sugar, raw sugar, date sugar, corn syrup, and honey

* Artificial sweeteners (like Aspartame and NutraSweet)

* Yeast containing foods - breads, pastries, and crackers

* Alcohol, soda, coffee, fermented drinks (like ciders)

* Malt containing products (such as malted milk drinks, cereals, candies)

* Condiments, salad dressings, sauces, vinegar containing foods (such as ketchup, mayonnaise, mustard, MSG and pickles)

* Dried and candied fruits (no raisins, dates, pineapple, etc.)

* Fermented foods (such as soy sauce, tofu, tempeh, sauerkraut)

* All fruit juice except all natural Granny Smith apples

* Cheese and sour milk products (such as buttermilk, sour cream)

* Mushrooms

* All nuts , except raw almonds

* Packaged, processed foods; including enriched flour products

No - No - No

Mustard

Ketchup

Worcestershire

Accent

Steak sauce

Barbecue sauce

Chili sauce

Soy sauce

Pickled anything

Relishes

Green olives

Sauerkraut

Horseradish

Mincemeat

Vinegar

Vinegar foods

Mayonnaise

Salad dressing

Malt products – all

Malted milk drinks

Malt cereals

Honey

Molasses

Maple syrup and sugar

Date sugar

Fruits and Fruit juice – all

Cheese – all

Yogurt

Bread – all

Pastries – all

Baked goods with yeast

"No No" – Sugar Foods - READ LABELS

Sugar
Corn syrup
White bread
White flour products
Sodas
Ready cereals
Roquefort * worst
Sweet Snack foods
Fat Snack foods

These are other names for sugar - Read Labels

Sucrose
Fructose
Maltose
Lactose
Glycogen
Glucose
Mannitol
Sorbitol
Galactose
Monosaccharide
Polysaccharides

Other No No Foods

Meats – smoked
Fish – pickled or smoked
Bacon, Ham, and Sausage
Hot dogs
Mushrooms
Corned beef
Pastrami
No Alcohol
No Beer, Wine
No Grains

The YES List

Foods You Can Eat

All fresh vegetables and vegetable juices – raw or cooked

All fish (except scavengers like catfish). Deep-sea white fish and salmon are the best.

Free Range chicken and turkey

Eggs

Drink 64 oz. of water a day!

Fresh lemon, lime, cranberries, Granny Smith apples, grapefruit. (Hint: any fruit that does not mold if left out of refrigerator)

Well-cooked whole grains: millet, buckwheat, amaranth, and quinoa. (No wheat)

Pasta made from any of the above grains

Essential fatty acids - one tablespoon per day of flax seed oil or flakes. Put flakes on salad.

Butter – not margarine

Grits but no corn

Beans (see list)

Raw almonds and seeds

Tea: chamomile, peppermint, Pau D'Arco

Green super foods are great to make smoothie. Such as Ultimate green, Barley green, Vital Green, green foods such as dried Spirulina. They can all be found at local health food store.

Sweetener: Stevia ONLY

Vegetables Choices -Cooked or Fresh

Asparagus
Artichoke
Avocado
Beets
Beet greens
Broccoli
Brussels sprouts
Cabbage
Carrots
Cauliflower
Celery
Chard, Swiss
Collard greens
Cucumbers
Daikon
Dandelion
Eggplant
Endive
Fennel
Garlic
Green pepper
Kale
Kohlrabi
Leeks
Lettuce – all kinds
Mustard greens
Okra
Onions
Parsley
Parsnips
Peas
Peppers, bell
Potatoes

Radishes
Rutabaga
Shallot
Snow Peas
Soybeans
Spinach
String beans
Squash, acorn/butternut
Tomatoes
Turnips

Meats - Eggs – Grains - Nuts -Seeds – Oil Choices

Fish
Salmon
Cod
Sardines
Mackerel
Tuna
Fresh fish
Frozen fish
Shrimp
Lobster
Crab
Seafood, other

Meat
Chicken
Turkey
Beef, lean
Veal
Lamb

Nuts, Seeds, Oils
Almonds
Brazil nuts
Cashews
Filbert
Flaxseeds
Pecans

Pumpkin seeds

<u>Cold Pressed Unrefined Oils</u>
Olive
Safflower
Sunflower
Soy
Walnut
Butter, real

<u>Grains</u>
Kamut a oriental wheat
Millet
Amarantha
Quinoa
Spelt
Rice
Buckwheat

MEAL SUGGESTIONS

Breakfast Choices

BREAKFAST because you have candida you cannot have fruit or fruit juice, because it turns to sugar. Therefore, I suggest a smoothie to hold you until noon, or some of the other breakfast suggestions below. You can have vegetable fruit in your smoothie. You can have a Granny Smith Apple. You can have "vegetable fruits" which are avocado, cucumbers, peppers, and tomatoes.

Drink EVERY MORNING for total DAILY fuel. This is designed to restore energy to your body by giving it the nutrition or fuel it needs to support your daily habits. Your car will not run without fuel and water, and neither will your body. Fatigue is a sign that you need nutrients.

Smoothie Breakfast Recipe in a blender #1
3 oz. Biomega (liquid vitamin see below)
Add 1-Granny Smith Apple
 Add 1 Tbs. SPN refresh (Potassium/Magnesium liquid minerals)
Add any approved veggies
1 tsp. Vitamin C powder (from Designs for health.com)
Blend and add ice

Smoothie Breakfast Recipe in a blender #2

4 oz to 1 cup Rice Dream Vanilla (from grocery store)

3 oz Biomega

1 oz SPN

1 Tsp. Vitamin C Powder w/MSM (from Designs for Health)

1 Tsp. Vitamin B Liquid (from Designs for Health)

2 Tbsp. Flax Powder from Fortifiedflax.com

ICE

You may add any or all of these

Granny Smith apples

Grapefruit

Carrots

Celery

Cucumbers

Parsley with any vegetables from yes food list

Other Breakfast Choices

Oatmeal with butter and/or flaxseed and pecans (Remember; make oatmeal from scratch not the just add water kind)

Brown rice with filberts and rice cakes.

Eggs with turkey bacon and grits with real butter

Amaranth cereal

Egg sandwich on no yeast or sour dough bread

Breakfast tacos

Omelet with raw veg.

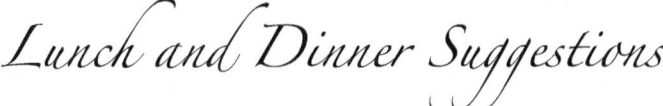

Lunch and Dinner Suggestions

* Soups with no corn or sugar

* Salmon on top of green salad with raw vegetables

* Salad Tuna fish w/lemon, celery, and pecans on lettuce

* Baked Cornish hens, steamed vegetables

* Steak cut on top of salad

* Hamburger patty on top of salad

* Roast turkey with steamed vegetables

Get the idea

You can do this

Put meals together from the list - It will make it easier

Remember carbs turn to sugar. Watch high carbs

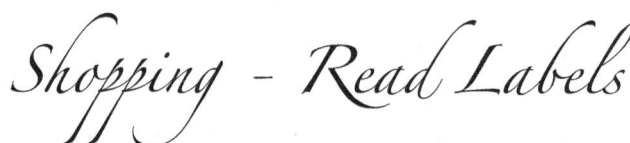

Shopping - Read Labels

Shop mainly around the outer edges of your market. Look for fresh and frozen vegetables, fresh meat, poultry, fish, seafood, eggs, olive oil, and pure butter. Try to buy organically grown foods if you can afford them. If not, make sure you wash them with a vegetable wash to eliminate pesticides and other chemical contaminates.

* Avoid foods labeled "enriched"

* Many canned, packaged and processed foods contain hidden ingredients, including sugar, and dextrose and other products. Avoid them.

* If you have no other choice and must use canned, read labels carefully

* If buying frozen vegetables, select those without added ingredients

**Avoid processed, smoked, or cured meats; they all contain sugar, spices, yeast, and other ingredients.

Surprise Foods THAT HAVE MOLD - Melons - Grapes - Corn

Replacements

Replace Sugar with: Stevia

It's an all-natural sweet herb that you can buy in granulated form, in little packets. It looks and tastes like sugar. You can sweeten with it, bake with it, and use it anywhere you would use sugar.

Use These Grains: amaranth, buckwheat, quinoa

You can find these in cereal form, or milled so you can bake with them. Find them with the prepared breads in the healthy section of your market. Try Flax Seed or Sunflower breads.

Very Very Very Important

Die Off and Detox

<u>YOU MUST MUST MUST Eliminate</u>

What is die off? Die off is the dead candida that you have killed from the program. It will gravitate to the colon. It should not stay in the body. You must eliminate it out of all system! It kinda looks like cottage cheese or string.

1. Flush it out with 64 oz of water a day, up to 1 gallon.

2. Sweat it out by exercise, steam room, sauna, and hot detox bath

* Eliminate it via requires bowel movements 3 times a day. Take a product to keep bowels moving daily as discussed earlier "Reneu". It is natural to have constipation when you have Candida and when you are taking Candistroy to kill it.

* Add fiber to your daily diet. It's easy,-just add 1-2 tablespoons of flax seed

powder or oil to your salad daily.

FATIGUE

Plan when you will start your detox. I suggest to begin when you have two days of nothing scheduled. The day you begin the *Candistroy* product, you will be very tired, remember a symptom the product is working is fatigue. The fatigue is a result of die off, the product is killing off the candida. Your body makes you tired so you will rest while it goes to work.

Remember, you do not want dead candida to stay in your body. Try to do activities to make you sweat:

1. try using a steam room

2. hot baths

3. sauna

4. walk rapidly, do a 15 minute mile

5. skin brush - brush you skin to open the lymph nodes

and most of all eliminate (bowel movements) several times a day. That is how the candida is excreted from the body.

If you are constipated, use "Reneu" 2 cap's every night.

Fungus die-off involves symptoms you will experience during the detoxification process of killing the candida

- Headaches
- Nausea
- Brain fog
- Dizziness

- Fatigue
- Sugar cravings
- Minor skin breakouts
- Cold hands and feet

Try not to take anything to cover these symptoms up. Ride them out; they will pass.

These are temporary, positive signs that the program is working.

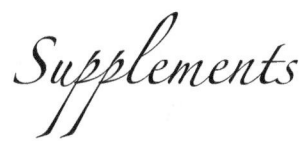

Supplements

We have discussed several of these previously, so this is a review.

Vitamins and minerals in liquid form
www.drklemere.firstfitness.com
Biomega is a liquid multi-vitamin in a aloe vera base.

SPN is a liquid Potassium/Magnesium.

Essential fatty acids: Use flax seeds or olive oil
Whole Food Grocery or Vitamin shop
Suggest:Omega Life, Inc. Fortified Flax seed powder or Barlenes Flax powder or oil

at market.

Vitamin C powder
Suggest: www.designsforhealth.com

Water:
Suggest: reverse osmosis

Probiotics
Suggest: "Healthy Trinity" by Natrin at Whole Foods or Amazon online

Other Supplements: CoQ10, Ginkgo biloba, Echinacea, Bromelain, grape seed
extract, Caprylic Acid, Citrus Seed Extract (Tricycline), Garlic, Goldenseal,
Colloidal Silver, Herbal Tea: Pau D' Arco, Peppermint, clover and Kombucha tea
contains many of the B vitamins to boost energy and improve the immune response
while you are detoxing.

Resource for Liquid Vitamins: *Biomega* from FirstFitness Nutrition
(drklemere.firstfitness.com distributor #11901)

Resources for liquid minerals: *SPN* from FirstFitness Nutrition
(drklemere.firstfitness.com distributor #11901)

Resources for Vitamin C power
www.designsforhealth.com

Eating Out - Choices

Breakfast: Vegetable omelet , no bread

Lunch: Vegetarian plate, Soup, Sour Dough sandwich

Dinner: Meat and salad combo (like the Steak Salad at Salt Grass)

Remember no salad dressing. Order olive oil, no vinegar, and fresh lemon, or bring your own. Anne's makes all natural salad dressing you can eat.

Restaurants

Mexican: Fajitas

Italian: Vegetable pasta (spinach pasta or other approved grain)

Seafood: Many choices

Luby's Cafeteria

Furr's Cafeteria

Cracker Barrel

Black Eyed Pea

Mimi's

ZuZu

Tips

* Have your meals list with you always.

* Use the list when ordering out, or cooking at home.

* Go with an idea of what you are going to eat

* Do not look at the menu and try to choose what is on the list.

* Know what to order ahead of time.

Do not look at the menu; have someone else order for you from your list.

Allergies

Often, allergies to food are present in people with Candida infections. The foods you crave or eat the most, are usually the foods to which you are allergic. Wheat, sugar, mayo, or ranch dressing (buttermilk) are major offenders. The symptoms of a food allergy or environmental sensitivity can also mimic those of Candidiasis. To further complicate matters, some people with Candidiasis go on to develop environmental sensitivities as well. Many cannot tolerate contact with or the smell of rubber, petroleum products, tobacco, exhaust fumes, or chemical odors.

When I first got sick, one of the first symptoms I experienced was during shopping. I could not shop anywhere near the tire department without becoming nauseated, dizzy, and my tongue going numb. I had to leave quickly or I would start a nosebleed. Thank goodness that over with! This is environmental sensitivity and not allergies. It is a symptom of poor health.

My clients are asked to make a commitment to follow the program for 8-12 weeks to eliminate the candida. I believe it will take a minimum of 90 days up to six months of treatment for the body to completely kill and eliminate candida, therefore cleansing itself down to the cellular level.

The Master Cleanser

Each system in your body requires a length of time to repair itself. For example, the intestinal lining repairs and replaces itself every three to five days. Before a system can repair or replace itself, it must have time out, giving the system a chance to rest without working. We accomplish this by using detoxification methods and cleansing. The best method is the master cleanse, which is a 10-day fasting without food. There are several different ways to fast; the master cleanse is by far the most difficult but the best. The majority of people find it hard to do the master cleanse because food has become such a source of comfort to combat stress.

A cleanse is used to detoxify your body and to cleanse your entire digestive system. The first four days of any cleanse that involves removing food is tough, but after the fourth day, you are no longer hungry. Before cleansing, I recommend preparing yourself and your body weeks in advanced. Slowly cut down on food. It is important to learn food choices and cooking methods that will work with your lifestyle and Candida detox program. The master cleanse is a kick start method for those who are seriously ill.

The purpose of the master cleanser is to dissolve and eliminate toxins and congestion that have formed in any part of the body. It is to purify the glands and cells throughout the entire body. It will cleanse the kidneys and the digestive system. It will eliminate all unusable waste including hardened material in the joints and muscles. It will relieve pressure and irritation in the nerves, arteries, and blood vessels. Then it will build a healthy blood stream. To accomplish this it will take 40 days.

It is best to follow the master cleanse for a minimum of 10 days up to 40 days (extremely serious cases can extend beyond 40 days). The diet has all the nutrition needed during this time. It is best to repeat the program at 4 times a year to keep the body in a healthy condition. Do not take any supplement during this time.

Mixing the Lemonade Cleanse in a 2 Quart container

Mix together in a 2 quart container
4 oz organic lemon or lime juice squeeze fresh
4 oz genuine maple syrup, Grade C or B if you can't find C
3 capsules cayenne pepper or to taste
Distilled or Spring Water filled to top of container

Peel 3 ORGANIC lemons. Put peeled lemons in a juicer to extract juice. Collect juice in a measuring cup. The 3 lemons should equal 4 oz. Pour 4 oz of lemon juice in a 2 quart container. *DO NOT USE A BLENDER TO MIX*

Add 4 oz of GRADE B or C maple syrup to lemon juice. The maple syrup you buy in most grocery stores is grade A and does not have the nutrients you need. The maple syrup has a balance of positive and negative sugar and can not be substituted. It also has a large variety of minerals and vitamins: Sodium, Potassium, Calcium, Magnesium, Manganese, Iron, Copper, Phosphorus, Sulphur, Chlorine, and Silicon, plus Vitamins. A, B1, B2, B6, C, and Nicotinic acid and Pantothenic acid. You can blend a part of the lemon skin and pulp with the lemonade.

Add Cayenne Pepper. Note: Cayenne is in the herb section in capsule form. Open 3 capsules and add to the lemon juice, add 4 if you have joint pain or stiffness. If you have burning with the Cayenne start with 1 capsule and build up to the 4 within 5 days.

Fill the balance of the 2 Qt. container with spring or distilled water. Stir well(do not put in a blender to mix). This mixture is your days supply of nutrition. Don't wait until you are hungry to drink your nutrition. Keep sipping all day and evening. You may make a second batch if you feel hungry. I drink mine in a 1 qt. jug with a straw. Drink 1 jug of lemonade, then a jug full of water, continue to rotate until all gone. Take with you in a cooler or refrigerator it to keep it cold and fresh all day. You can also drink it hot. Do not mix the night before, the mixture loses the nutritional benefit after sitting all night.

Do not eat ANY food or take ANY supplements while on this liquid diet. It takes about 3 days to settle into this routine. Your mind is programmed to eat meals and it takes awhile to break this thought process.

Prepare to do this for a minimum of 10 days. To receive the full benefits, you really need to plan to do it for the full 40 days. The longer you go the better you will feel. (you didn't get this way in 10 days) Try for the full 40 days. I did it for 40+ days and felt like a new person. The longer you can stay on this, the better you will feel. About day 7 all your joint pain and stiffness should be gone and you have a lot of energy.

You will loose weight. Most of my clients have lost 25 lb. in 40 days. If you don't want to lose weight just add more maple syrup, this will keep your weight up.

In the beginning as your body begins to detox, you will have a lot more stuff to eliminate. I suggest starting on a Saturday morning so over the weekend you can be at home. By Monday you will have the bathroom routine down and will have eliminated the bulk of the stuff you have been stuffing into your colon all these years. If you do not begin to eliminate the first day, you must something to open the systems up. Drink salt water really hot in the morning and evening is an easy way to get things moving. Most clients have to take the salt water 2 days. Your colon has a clean passage when you eliminate 30 minutes after eating a meal. This is the sign of a healthy colon Note: You should have at least 4 bowel movements a day. The better the elimination process, the more rapid the results. A laxative herb tea should be taken the last thing at night and the first thing in the morning.You can drink lax tea in the evening or take Reneu. You can buy a special blend of lax tea from the market in the herbal tea section. You need this to allow the Lymphatic system to rest and to deep cleanse the elimination organs. Mint tea may be used. Its chlorophyll helps as a purifier, neutralizing many mouth and body odors that are released during the cleansing period.

REMEMBER:

Jesus Christ fasted and prayed for 40 days. Men and Women fast for spiritual enlightenment, YOU CAN DO IT!

AT THE END OF YOUR lemonade cleanse, you must come off the diet as follows:

1st and 2nd day:

Drink four to six 8 oz glasses of fresh orange juice made in your juicer, as desired during the day

2nd day

Drink four to six 8 oz of orange juice during the day with add water for sensitive stomachs.

Prepare the following soup for dinner:

Organic: legumes, potatoes, celery, carrots, green vegetable tops, onion and Dehydrated vegetable soup powder for extra flavor. Okra or okra powder, chili, curry, cayenne pepper, tomatoes, green peppers and zucchini squash may be included for nutritional taste good advantage. Brown rice may be used, but no meat or meat stock. Other spices may be added for flavor. Use salt separately. The less cooking the better.

3rd day

Orange juice in the morning

Fresh raw fruit for lunch

Salad with fresh fruit and raw vegetable for dinner

<u>4th day</u>

Normal healthy eating may be resumed

In Conclusion

Having energy and being able to think clearly is a desired way of life at any age. The nutritional program designed in this little book will help children suffering from overweight and fatigue to senior adults with daily fatigue. I have used this program on my clients with great success for years and I have seen fantastic results. I encourage you to stick with the program, do not quit. The biggest mistake people make is quitting as soon as they start feeling better. In a month, the fungus returns vigorously, so do not quit.

A tip for success is to pick a time to start. If you work, start on a Friday. Do not plan to do the program over a holiday such as Thanksgiving, Christmas, or New Years.

Remember, ninety days to health!

Blessings of Health

Kay B. LeMere, N.D., Ph.D.

Let me hear about your experience contact me at:

www.author-kblemere.com